Beautifully Made!

Wisdom from a Woman:
Mother's Guide
(Book 3)
Second Edition

Edited by
Julie Hiramine

GENERATIONS OF VIRTUE

Scripture quotations are taken from The Holy Bible, New King James Version Copyright © 1982 by Thomas Nelson, Inc. and The Holy Bible, New International Version Copyright © 1978 by New York International Bible Society.

Contributors:

Julie Hiramine	Mary Whitlock
Sara Raley	Beth Lockhart
Annie Anderson	Chris McCausland
Megan Briggs	Kelsey McCausland

Artwork: Anne Brandenburg
All contributions were made as a free-will gift to Generations of Virtue

Beautifully Made! Wisdom from a Woman: Mother's Guide
Copyright © 2003 by Generations of Virtue
Second Edition © 2005 by Generations of Virtue

Published by: Generations of Virtue
P.O. Box 62253
Colorado Springs, CO 80962
www.generationsofvirtue.org

ISBN: 978-0-9766143-2-6

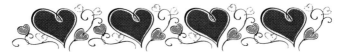

Table of Contents

www.generationsofvirtue.org
"Purity of Heart, Purity of Mind, Purity of Body"

They are all plain to him who understands,
And right to those who find knowledge.

Receive my instruction, and not silver,
And knowledge rather than choice gold;

For wisdom is better than rubies,
And all the things one may desire cannot be com-
pared with her.

I, wisdom, dwell with prudence,
And find out knowledge and discretion.

Proverbs 8:9-12

Foreword

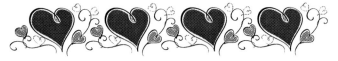

I have a heart to help moms deal with the changes their daughters go through as they reach adolescence. As I began to look for resources about starting menstruation that Generations of Virtue could carry to help parents meet their daughters' needs, I was appalled at how inappropriate the most popular books were. To this date I have not found a book that I would be confident in giving my daughter. The books I read were inappropriate to give to a girl who had her eyes set on virtue and purity. This celebration of womanhood is not a celebration of our daughters having compromising values, but a celebration of how God has created us as women. Many of us were not raised to see this as a celebration. I feel this is a time to change this negative thinking with the next generation. This book is meant to be used in conjunction with the first two books in the series that we wrote for daughters, entitled <u>Approaching Womanhood</u> and <u>Celebrating Womanhood</u>.

Julie Hiramine

Mothers Are the Experts

> You shall teach them diligently to your children, and shall talk of them when you sit in your house, when you walk by the way, when you lie down, and when you rise up.
> Deuteronomy 6:7[1]

There have been days as a mother that I have wondered if I am an expert about anything, especially all the changes my daughters are going through. Then God speaks and confirms that He is the One who has given me these precious children as gifts and equipped me to be their guide for this season. Now this book for moms is meant to show our daughters how we can celebrate the gifts God has given us as women. Almost all the moms I have talked with did not have any celebration.

1. All scriptures are taken from the New King James Version (NKJV) of the Bible.

Once I read a story that went something like this: Wouldn't your life have been different if, on the day you started your period, your mom gave you flowers and took you to lunch?[1] I think my view of myself and menstruation would have been very different if there had been a celebration at this key rite of passage.

The first principle I want to stress to moms is that God has appointed and commissioned you to be the expert for your children in the areas of sex education and virtue. Although you might need to be equipped, you are the person that God has chosen to give your children the critical information they will need to chart the future course for their lives. This is the season when you pour yourself out and fill them with godly wisdom and understanding. This is important to do from the time they are young.

1. Northrup, Christiane. <u>Women's Bodies, Women's Wisdom</u>. Bantam Books: New York, 1998. Page 101

No one can take your place. No teacher, "expert," pastor, or counselor can take the place of moms and dads who love their children like no one else. Others cannot be there at those moments when your kids ask all kinds of probing questions that are so spontaneous. Only you know the special needs of your children and how each child is different. Your daughter can sit while a supposed expert addresses a mass audience, but that message will not be as personalized as the one you give your child. Please know that you are the one to whom God has assigned this significant task, and it is you who will accomplish it the very best.

Is Now the Time?

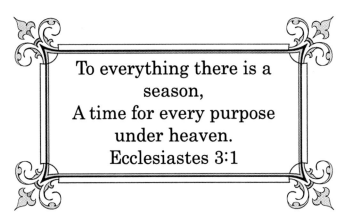

To everything there is a
season,
A time for every purpose
under heaven.
Ecclesiastes 3:1

Now, to get to the pertinent topic at hand: talking with our daughters. When is the best time to talk with our daughters about menstruation and the changes they will go through as they approach adolescence? Usually between the ages of eight and ten is the peak time to talk with them. Remember that you are the very best person that God has ordained to provide this critical information to your daughter.

I remember one day at my hairdresser's. She was cutting away, and we were talking about our daughters when the subject of their maturing came up. As she cut my hair, I can recall a sense of dread setting over me as she said, "You know, girls start their periods two

9

years earlier then we did." I started doing the math...I started my period when I was 11, and my daughter is 8. That means she could start as early as 9 years old! Ahhhhh! I better get my act together.

It is better to talk with our daughters and prepare them even if they seem like our "little girls." They need to be equipped. Another reason to talk with them, even if it seems early, is to avoid the possibility that the neighbor girl down the street will be the first one to talk to them about this subject. If some other child tells them, their facts will probably not be correct, and it will not be coming from one of the people who love them most.

Teachable Moments…Opening the Lines of Communication

> *Happy is the man who finds wisdom,*
> *And the man who gains understanding.*
> *Proverbs 3:13*

The key to talking with our daughters when they are young is in the "teachable moment." When I say "moment," I mean it. Catch those moments while you are driving or making dinner when spontaneous questions can arise. It doesn't have to be a long discourse with planned diagrams, but a few moments of well-placed wisdom. Many times the attention span of our daughters is in and out. These seeds are being planted to grow for continual discovery. Plant seeds every chance you get. Girls at this age cannot grasp the entire picture of menstruation in just one sitting. It takes many times of explaining in a myriad of ways for our daughters to feel confident about this complicated process.

It is also important, along with these "teachable moments," to have a longer discus- 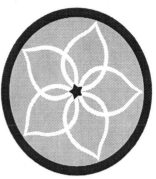 sion with all the facts presented. The book Approaching Woman- hood is a great resource to sit down and review with your daughter. Our girls will have an entire gamut of differ- ent responses in this time with us. Some will act disinterested and look away, while others will be shocked and surprised by the details of this process. Press on and share with them in a positive manner. Also, try to remember anything about which you can speak posi- tively from your own experience. If you can't think of anything positive, you might say, "When I started my period, I was so shocked it frightened me. This is why I want to share with you all these things so you will be much more prepared than I was. You can always talk with me about this and feel free to ask me any questions about this."

Leading Predictors

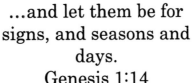

...and let them be for
signs, and seasons and
days.
Genesis 1:14

There are several predictors associated with puberty for moms to watch for as their daughters mature. These signs will alert you that your daughter is approaching menses. Don't wait until all of these have happened or it might be too late!

First, breasts begin to develop with a slight elevation and then continue to grow. Sometimes each breast does not grow at the same rate; this is perfectly normal. The next indicator is that pubic and armpit hair begin to grow. Another sign is that their 12-year molars come in. Lastly, there is a growth spurt right before the start of their periods that includes both weight gain and an increase in height. Normally they grow taller first, and then about six months later they begin to gain weight.

With gladness and rejoicing
they shall be brought;
They shall enter the King's
palace.
Psalm 45:15

Although our moms did not give us a cause to celebrate when we started our periods, it can be very different for our own daughters. As I noted earlier in this book, it would have been so different for us if our mothers had celebrated with us by taking us to lunch and giving us flowers. For me, it would have made the moment memorable in a positive way rather than distressing. Think back to when you started your period. What was the response of those around you? What were your own feelings like? How would you like this experience to be different for your daughter?

Starting menstruation has been a rite of passage in many cultures, including the Jewish culture. This has somehow been lost for the most part in our high-tech world. Now can be a time to recapture a little of this great tradition. It can be a time for celebration and a time to foster communication between a mother and her daughter.

Here are a few ideas and suggestions that may get you started thinking about a creative way to celebrate your daughter's menses. The first one I have shared already. It is to have a special lunch together and buy her a bouquet of flowers. During this special lunch time, share about your experience and confirm to her the beauty of God's timing and His plan for her life.

Another thing you could do is get her ears pierced. Then maybe Dad could meet you both at the jewelry store and buy a special pair of earrings that represent her commitment to purity and virtue. Some girls don't want their dads to know that they started their periods and are embarrassed. Use your best judgment.

This could open the door for fathers and daughters to communicate openly about these issues. It is also great for a daughter to know that her dad cares and that the process of her becoming a woman is one he embraces. If dads are involved all the way along in this process, it will be easier for daughters to approach them for wisdom and advice as the years go by.

Another idea is for you to get a special journal in which your daughter could record her feelings. You could also write a special letter affirming the work God is doing in her life as she approaches womanhood and how exciting it is.

Another approach is to take your daughter to a special concert or to hear the symphony. It is an offer to do something special with Mom and Dad that is a bit more grown-up. A special dinner could be the prelude to the concert.

A special brunch for your daughter, to which significant women in her life are invited, such as grandmothers, older sisters, aunts, and others, can be a special way to celebrate. They can share stories, insight, and wisdom with her during this time.

Going together to buy supplies and toiletries may be a fun outing together. Be sure to have a variety of pads and supplies on hand at home as well, even before she starts. Do not assume that the products you use will work for her. She is still smaller than you and needs her own supplies. She might need shaving cream and a razor if she hasn't already begun to shave. One family I know bought special "period underwear" for their daughter to wear during her period. That way she doesn't stain and ruin her favorite cute underwear. You could go together to shop for these necessary supplies.

A day at the spa together as mother-daughter to get a manicure and have lunch is another way to celebrate.

Another idea is to purchase a special purity ring or necklace and put it away for when her period starts. Mother and Father can give that to her as a symbol of the time of maturing she is now entering.

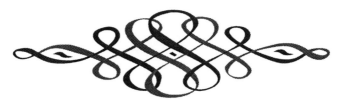

Any activity to celebrate and help your daughter feel more grown-up is appropriate for this time. There are so many ideas to do together. Most importantly, any kind of activity together should build the lines of communication and celebrate the start of a new phase of life. When this phase is entered into positively, it can impact her future concept of what it means that God made her a woman.

Your Daughter's Changing Moods

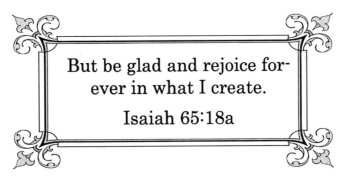

But be glad and rejoice for-
ever in what I create.

Isaiah 65:18a

When your daughter's period starts, there will be lots of ups and downs. Recognizing these patterns can be very helpful in relating to your daughter. In the book <u>The Wonder of Girls</u>, author Michael Gurian includes wonderful insight into the world of hormones and chemicals that work in your daughter's life.

His explanation of brain chemistry and hormones is incredibly helpful to understand the ways God created our inner workings. The passage I would like to share with you, set in italics below, is about how hormones affect your daughter's monthly cycle.

Stage 1: The First Half. Weeks one and two of her monthly cycle.

Estrogen and endorphin levels are gradually rising. Her mood is relatively stable, even upbeat, as they rise. Serotonin, dopamine, norepinephrine, and other nerve cells that regulate mood are high in response to high estrogen and endorphin levels. She might be doing pretty well on her math tests, her reading, and other academic skills. She might be living with a certain amount of ease.

Stage 2: Midcycle. Around two weeks before her period begins.

Estrogen levels shoot up, then drop suddenly. This is a trauma to the brain, which goes into a kind of withdrawal. Your daughter may experience a lot of things we listed [including mood disruptions, anxiousness, lack of concentration, drop in self-esteem, feelings of being overwhelmed, angry outbursts, hypersensitivity, self-criticism, energy depletion, and increased irritability].

This withdrawal—a "down" mood, "she's quieter than usual," "she's moody"—can be even more pronounced in certain girls because of two factors: genetic predisposition and/or external stress. Many girls are predisposed to

more or less difficulty at certain times of the cycle.

If your daughter is predisposed to more difficulty in mood regulation during Stage 2, she may confuse you during this time especially. She "may not be herself." Her self-esteem may plummet.

At some point in life most if not all girls and women go through some kind of difficulty in Stage 2 mood regulation. And most go through some measure of it every month. It is part of a female's journey through life.

If she is under a lot of stress (or has been experiencing accumulated trauma, from abuse of some kind or from a divorce or broken relationship), she may also experience severe mood swings during this time. She may do less well in school, lose her focus, and experience a number of things we listed.

Stage 3: Ovulation and Post-Ovulation.

Ovulation is such a "positive trauma" to the nerve cells, that the fog often lifts as quickly as it came. Now estrogen levels begin to rise again. Progesterone levels also rise, reaching their peak about seven to eight days after

33

ovulation, then declining over the next few days. Rising progesterone is a mood-stabilizing influence on the brain: Progesterone attaches to GABA receptors (that quiet the brain) and interacts with serotonin to create feelings of wellness. This is a great time to be a girl!

Testosterone levels gradually rise during the female cycle, becoming highest toward the end of midcycle/beginning of ovulation.

Stage 4: The Final Days.

Estrogen drops, followed by progesterone and the endorphins. What may have been experienced in Stage 2 can be even more amplified in your daughter in Stage 4. The sweet, even wonderful feelings of high self-esteem and readiness to face the world experienced by your daughter in Stage 3 can disappear in Stage 4.

The brain deals with the traumas of falling estrogen, progesterone, and endorphins by exhibiting anger, hypersensitivity, irritability, sadness, feelings of despair, and lowered self-esteem. It can seem like your daughter is forgetting things a lot; her food intake

may change, as she craves carbohydrates. She may hide in her room. You may really come to worry about her. She may well appear very depressed. Her brain is short-circuiting.[2]

This is part of the adventure of having girls. Their emotional makeup changes as different hormones are released from their brains. This affects some of our girls more than others. It is good to keep track of their cycles so we know how to respond to them at different times.

2. Gurian, Michael. *The Wonder of Girls*. Pocket Books: New York, 2002. Pages 83-84

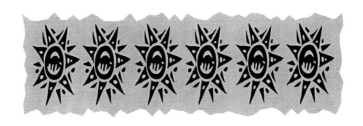

Biology

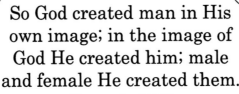

> So God created man in His
> own image; in the image of
> God He created him; male
> and female He created them.
> Genesis 1:27

Menstrual Cycle

The menstrual cycle is composed of three phases: the menstrual flow phase, the proliferative phase, and the secretory phase.

Menstrual Flow Phase—this phase marks the beginning of the menstrual cycle. Day 1 of the cycle starts when bleeding occurs. During this time, the lining of the uterus sheds from the uterine wall. This phase lasts approximately three to five days.

Proliferative Phase—During this time, the remaining portion of the uterine lining begins to thicken and regenerate. This lasts about two to three weeks.

Secretory Phase—The uterine lining continues to thicken, meanwhile becoming more vascularized (blood vessels start to form). It also develops glands that secrete a fluid rich in glycogen (a sugar). This lasts about two weeks. If an embryo is planted in the uterine lining before the end of the secretory phase, the menstrual cycle stops in order for the uterus to harbor a child. However, if no embryo is present in the lining at the end of the secretory phase, the menstrual cycle starts over with the menstrual flow phase.

Ovarian Cycle

The ovarian cycle consists of two phases: the follicular phase and the luteal phase. These phases are momentarily disrupted by ovulation, which is the release of a not quite completed egg cell.

Follicular Phase- A follicle consists of one developing egg cell surrounded by one or more layers of follicle cells, which function in nourishing and protecting the egg cell. Follicles are located in the ovaries. During the follicular phase, the egg cell begins to enlarge inside each follicle, and its layer of follicle cells thickens. However, only one follicle usually continues to enlarge and mature while the others disintegrate. The maturing follicle develops an internal, fluid-filled cavity and grows very large, forming a bulge near the surface of the ovary. Ovulation marks the end of the follicular phase, as the follicle and adjacent wall of the ovary rupture, releasing the developing egg cell.

Luteal Phase- The follicular tissue that remains in the ovary becomes the corpus luteum, which secretes additional estrogens and progesterone during pregnancy. These hormones help regulate the uterine lining so that a developing embryo can remain stable. It is also important to note that an egg cell has not completed its development until it is fertilized with a sperm cell.

43

If the egg cell is not fertilized, the corpus luteum dissolves.

Hormones

Hormones coordinate the menstrual and ovarian cycles so that an egg cell is released when it will be able to be planted in the uterine lining. Hormones regulate the ovarian and menstrual cycles so that an egg cell is released during the secretory phase of the menstrual cycle. This ensures that the egg cell meets appropriate conditions in order to be fertilized and start developing. In other words, if an egg cell was released during the menstrual phase of the menstrual cycle, the egg cell could not attach to the uterine wall because the lining would not be there, or it would be in the process of shedding. Another important fact is that in order to support life, the uterine wall must be vascularized by the time the egg cell attaches to it so that the egg cell will have a means of discarding waste and receiving vital nutrients such as oxygen and glucose from the blood. Without these means, the egg cell could not divide into tissues and eventually a baby because cells require several materials like water, oxygen, and glucose in order to undergo mitosis (cell division).

45

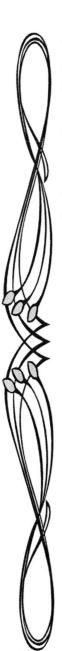

The hormones involved in the menstrual and ovarian cycles are: gonadotropin-releasing hormone (GnRH), secreted by the hypothalamus (which is part of the brain); follicle-stimulating hormone (FSH), secreted by the anterior pituitary (also in the brain); luteinizing hormone (LH), which is also secreted by the anterior pituitary; estrogens (which are a group of closely related hormones), secreted by the ovaries; and progesterone, also secreted by the ovaries.

In a nutshell, these hormones function as follows: the hypothalamus basically controls when and to what extent the hormones estrogen and progesterone are released. The hormones secreted from the brain (GnRH, FSH, LH) coordinate the menstrual and ovarian cycles, while the hormones from the ovaries (estrogens and progesterone) regulate the actual functions in the ovaries and uterus.

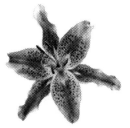

Counsel is mine, and
sound wisdom; I am
understanding, I have
strength.
Proverbs 8:14

For mothers, I recommend calling
your daughter's teacher and explaining her situation. This will greatly
reduce her stress and really put her at
ease knowing that someone can help
her when you are not around. This
way, her teacher can be sensitive about
bathroom trips, cramping, etc. I recommend buying a small, purse-like
container in which to put feminine
products so that she can discreetly
take tampons and/or pads to the rest-
room. If she is using pads, try find-
ing thin ones that will work and that
she can keep in a back pocket.
Kelsey, 18 years old

A natural supplement we have found to work well if you are having problems with your period or cramping is Evening Primrose Oil or Total EFA Flaxseed Oil, which has Evening Primrose Oil in it. This product can be found at a health foods store. The best way to take this is in its oil form. If you find you don't like the taste of the oil, you can disguise it in flavored yogurt.

Another area that can cause our daughters stress is going to a sleepover or off to camp. Make sure she is comfortable with what to do in these situations. Talk about your daughter's concerns with other moms or counselors who will be with her. This is mainly a problem when girls are younger and do not want everyone to know that they have started their period. As girls grow older they will begin to discuss their period among their friends and not be so embarrassed by the subject.

Help your daughter, as well, with the use of tampons if swimming is one of the activities in which she will be participating. Encourage her to try again if her first try is not successful.

When she does start wearing tampons, have her consider wearing a pad with them until she gets used to how long she can wait before she changes them.

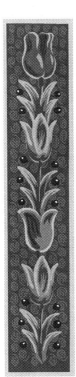

A few words about toxic shock syndrome (TSS): It is important that pubescent girls only wear tampons for activities when they are necessary (like swimming) and that they change them every four hours. Do not use "super" high absorbency tampons at this age. It is vital that our daughters realize that when using a tampon the vagina is an abundant breeding ground for bacteria and that tampons need to be changed regularly. Our daughters need to let adults around them know they are wearing tampons in case they start exhibiting symptoms of TSS.

Symptoms of toxic shock syndrome are as follows: fever over 102 degrees, faintness or dizziness, diarrhea, nausea or vomiting, and a sunburn-like rash that is painless. This is an issue that we need to make our daughters aware of because it can be very serious, even life threatening.

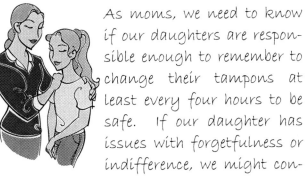

As moms, we need to know if our daughters are responsible enough to remember to change their tampons at least every four hours to be safe. If our daughter has issues with forgetfulness or indifference, we might consider not allowing her to wear tampons until she is more responsible.

Go with your daughter to buy supplies and pick the kind of pads she wants to wear. Have her try them on and do some of her normal activities so that she gets used to wearing a pad and knows what to do with them before her period even starts. Also, it is a good idea to buy your daughter her own deodorant and remind her to wear it every day.

Go over with your daughter what to do if her pad leaks onto her clothes or if she leaks at night onto her sheets. Help her know how to handle these situations if she is at a friend's house or at a sleepover.

Of all these ideas, the most important is to keep the lines of communication open. Let her know that you are there to listen to her concerns and feelings that surround these issues.

Personal Experience

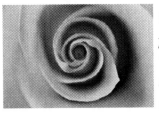

We are a family of four girls and one boy. Three of the girls have been on the journey to womanhood for quite awhile now. As mom, I will try and pass on some of the things I have learned from our journey. As I remember it, each girl did very well with that first experience. They all three included me in the day but also wanted privacy and for me not to "run and call my friends."

The biggest adjustments in the months ahead were mood swings and cramps. The mood swings were noticed right away. That is a tough balance as a parent. You want to be understanding and yet not make it an excuse for sin. Being aware of your daughter's cycle is helpful, though at first it can be unpredictable. An extra amount of patience, kindness, gentleness, etc, can go a long way that week before. Yet I think it would be helpful to stress that it is not an excuse for extreme anger and emotion.

There are so many good resources on the Internet these days that would help. Diet seems to be a good place to start looking to see if what they are eating could be affecting the dreaded PMS! Exercise is also very important.

Cramps are another issue that would be good to research. We have tried everything from heating pads, to mild pain killers, to birth control pills for one daughter. I do not recommend birth control pills. She was very irregular and had bad cramps, and it was recommended by doctors that we put her on them. After that experience, we recommend natural remedies as opposed to traditional methods.

My middle child, who is now 18, started when she was 10. It was not at all surprising to me because she had shown signs of puberty at an early age. The adjustment was slightly more difficult for her.

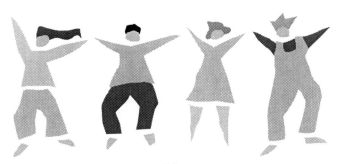

Being sensitive to her
needs, such as phoning her
teacher and being discreet
around her friends, was
very important to her. I encourage all mothers to talk
with their daughters about
their needs during this
special time.
And on a lighter note, our
house is now a tampon
drugstore. Be ready to try
lots of different kinds of
feminine products in all
shapes and sizes. Your
daughter may not find the
perfect product for some
time, but comfort is important and needs to be taken
into consideration.
-Chris, Mother of 5

61

A Word About Generations of Virtue

The ministry of Generations of Virtue believes God is raising this current generation to be godly men and women with pure hearts, minds, and bodies. We long to see our society become one that worships God with its whole being. Our vision is that of a generation that does not look to meaningless, vain relationships for comfort. We long to see a generation that calls to God to be its number one adviser and guardian. This goal, we believe, is to be attained through the help of parents. For this reason, Generations of Virtue provides parents and teens with the counsel and resources they need to discover God's gift of purity and His promise to be the protector of our love lives.

Generations of Virtue does not simply promote abstinence. We believe in the merits of courtship and the importance of emotional, spiritual, and physical purity. If you are looking for resources to teach your children about God's design for romance and relationships, or if you are a teen looking to find the truth about purity, we invite you to take a look at our website and the resources we offer. Generations of Virtue is an up-and-coming organization, so look for new additions as we grow.

www.generationsofvirtue.org

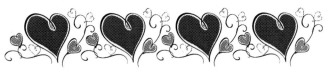

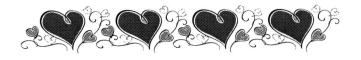

If you enjoyed this book, please check out
the other books in the
Beautifully Made! Series-

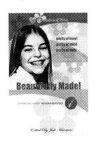

Approaching Womanhood- This is the first book
in the *Beautifully Made!* series, designed for
mother-daughter discussion and bonding time.
Help your daughter through this potentially
stressful experience while she anticipates her first
period. This book is designed to encourage your
daughter as it discusses issues all developing
girls face and wonder about: her changing body,
her first period, her body image, and how she can
be prepared if her period starts unexpectedly, and,
most importantly, her worth in God's eyes and
her role in God's kingdom.
Recommended for girls ages 8-12.

www.generationsofvirtue.org
"Purity of Heart, Purity of Mind, Purity of Body"

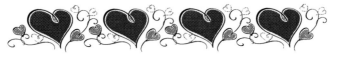

Celebrating Womanhood: Book 2 in the Beautifully Made! Series-

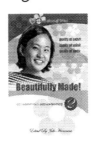

Celebrating Womanhood- Having your period is something to celebrate, and this booklet explains why. The second book in the *Beautifully Made!* series, *Celebrating Womanhood* covers subjects like "PMS", which products to use and how to use them, tips on health, and much more. You and your daughter can share quality mother-daughter time as you read and discuss this book; afterward, she can keep the booklet as a continuous reference. Biblically centered, this book will give your daughter an encouraging message about her period. **Recommended as a gift for your daughter at the start of her first period.**

www.generationsofvirtue.org
"Purity of Heart, Purity of Mind, Purity of Body"

If you enjoyed this resource please order these other recommended resources found on our website.

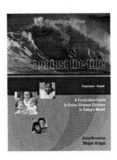

Against the Tide Elementary Guide

By
Julie Hiramine and Megan Briggs

Age-appropriate training for young ones!

God calls His people to be set apart from the world; He calls us to be sanctified. In an effort to accomplish this requirement, Julie Hiramine and Megan Briggs have organized a curriculum guide for the preschool to fourth grade years designed to train your children in purity and to solidify the process of character development. *Against the Tide— Elementary* is a year-by-year guide covering the basics of where babies come from, modesty, manners, and character development through assignments from resources Generations of Virtue feels are beneficial for young children. This guide focuses on building a solid foundation for the road to adulthood with age-appropriate character building and sex education.

Against the Tide Middle School Guide

By
Julie Hiramine and Megan Briggs

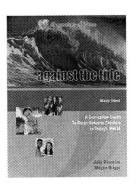

Practical Training for Preteens!

The 'tween years are a pivotal time in the shaping of your child's convictions, body image, relationship with figures of authority, and more. This curriculum guide is for 10- to 14-year olds and, like its predecessor for elementary-aged children, highlights when and how to use age-appropriate sex education and character training. *Against the Tide—Middle School* will help parents and children establish a practical approach to purity training. After reviewing hundreds of products, this guide will take you through the resources we have found to be most beneficial for young people. Also included with this guide are free updates every year in order to keep you posted on the new, up-to-date resources we have found after a year of searching. Take the leg-work out of establishing a purity-training plan with this excellent guide.

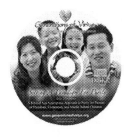

Setting A Paradigm For Purity—CD

By Julie Hiramine

Founder and Executive Director of Generations of Virtue, Julie Hiramine gives her biblically-centered and thoroughly researched advice regarding raising morally pure children. Mother of four girls, Julie shares her trials and triumphs concerning raising children in today's culture during her 90 minute discussion. On this CD, parents will learn what to talk about with their kids at every stage of development. Also included is information on how to set the paradigm for purity and courtship beginning in preschool, how parents can begin now to open the lines of communication in preparation for adolescence, and the art of media discernment.

Setting A Paradigm For Purity—DVD

By Julie Hiramine

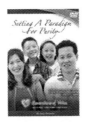

Filmed during a recent ministry trip to Asia, dynamic speaker **Julie Hiramine** addresses parents in Singapore with elementary- and middle school-aged children in this 90 minute discussion. Learn about training your children while they are young and most impressionable in this seminar for parents. Julie provides an age-appropriate plan for teaching your children about sex and virtuous character—two subjects that go hand in hand. You'll learn about the strategies necessary to guide your young one through the battlefield of today's culture as Julie addresses issues such as parental involvement and the impact it has on children, media discernment and how to teach it to your children, tools to use to set a courtship standard while your children are young, and simple ways to incorporate age-appropriate sex education that will empower your children and not burden them with too much or wrong information. God has designated you—the parents—as the experts for raising your children. Therefore, you want to be the ones to tell your children about sex, true love, and godly behavior. Don't wait until your child is a teenager and has already received and accepted a false message from the culture before you decide to train them. Directing your children into the path of holiness is not the impossible task you may think it is—especially when you incorporate the advice found on this DVD. Another feature included on the DVD is a segment which highlights other resources you can use with your children to teach them about and guide them to God's standard of purity.

AVAILABLE FOR THE FIRST TIME ON AUDIO CD!

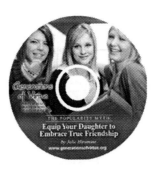

THE POPULARITY MYTH: Equip Your Daughter to Embrace True Friendship
by Julie Hiramine

Is your daughter the "odd girl out" or the "leader of the pack"? The rise and fall of the hierarchies of our daughters, and their siblings and friends, is like the rise and fall of kingdoms and world powers. How do we as parents deal with the cliques and their fall out? What is a Godly pattern for our girls and how should they structure their relationships? How do the lies of our culture perpetuate the need for our daughters to bolster their self image and define themselves through the eyes of their peers? Hear about God's design for our daughters and their relationships in this presentation. Step off the treadmill of our culture's say so and into the Spirit of God as the architect of relationships...even those of girls. **Recommended for mothers of girls**

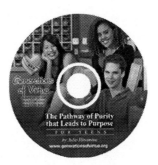